El Blackwood

Tending

Salamander Street

PLAYS

First published in 2024 by Salamander Street Ltd., a Wordville imprint. (info@salamanderstreetcom).

Tending © Eleanor Blackwood, 2024

Cover illustration by Eleanor Birdsall-Smith

ISBN: 9781068696220

10 9 8 7 6 5 4 3 2 1

Further copies of this publication can be purchased from www.salamanderstreet.com

Wordville

For every NHS nurse.

ACKNOWLEDGEMENTS

There is no one that has given more of themselves to this play than Izzy Howes. Thank you for not only being my best friend, but for being the inspiration for *Tending*. You are nothing short of extraordinary.

To every single nurse that contributed to *Tending*—thank you does not cover it. Thank you for trusting me with your stories, even when they were hard to talk about. Thank you for allowing me to listen to you, and trusting me to convey what it is to be a nurse. I have learned so much from you. Thank you as well for championing the play—giving up your time, energy and connections. It has been wonderful meeting so many of you in person, too, and the people close to you. While I've committed to anonymity for everyone interviewed, I would (with their permission) like to especially thank Duncan Lee and Sissi Serlenga. Thank you for putting me in touch with so many others, shouting about *Tending* from the rooftops, and being so supportive throughout this entire process.

To the people that brought *Tending* to life: Thank you to my brilliant creative partner, John Livesey. I am so grateful for your direction, dramaturgy and unparalleled artistic eye. You are nothing short of a slay. Ellie Birdsall-Smith, thank you for being truly fantastic, and never being phased despite the significant stresses that come with taking a show to the Fringe. Thank you to our Sound Designer, Sarah Spencer, and Lighting Designer Ros Chase for contributing their significant talent to create truly exceptional visual and aural worlds. Thank you to actors Stella Saltibus, Alasdair Linn, Ben Lynn and Mara Allen. Special thanks too to Philippa Lawford, Alex Rugman and Cam Spain, who gave up their time to offer insightful feedback. Lastly, thank you to John Burgess, who passed away before he could see this published. John's mentorship, guidance and—above all—friendship, is something that I'll treasure for the rest of my life.

There are also several organisations that have supported *Tending* along different phases of its journey. Thank you to the Clonterbrook Writer's Residency for giving me the space and time to write, and to Theatre Peckham for giving us space to rehearse. Thank you to Greenside Venues, Underbelly Edinburgh, and Brixton House. Thank you to the Tartan Silk Team for advocating for the show, and enabling us to share *Tending* with large audiences. Thank you to the Burdett Trust for

Nursing and the SIT-UP awards, for believing in the production enough to give us the financial support we needed to share it with audiences. And, to our phenomenal charity partner, Cavell Nurses' Trust. You do such exceptional work. Thank you also to the Salamander Street team, especially Lucy George, for believing in this script enough to publish it.

To the people who generously donated their own funds—I am so grateful. It was unbelievably kind and put simply, we wouldn't have been able to perform without you. This includes—but is in no way limited to!—Maggie Paterson, Harry Petty, Lili Momeni, Leo Benedict, Sophie Steyn, Elise O'Brien, Eimer McAuley, Chris Dodsworth, Jed Rubin, Danika Patel, Karen and Andrew Howes, Sue and Ritchie Hurst, Lizzette Robleto, Kevin Howarth, Danika Patel, James Pearson-Howes, Josephine Anderson, Tala Cingilioglu, Steve Rigby, Sarah Kidd, Mark Smith, Ruth Beal, Kerry Woodward-Fisher, Eddy Heylen, Cliff Calvert, Nicola Dinan, Eleanor Bowen, Chris Sheridan, Tara Jennett, Claire Lee and Brendan Beal.

Thank you to my mother and sisters, Debbie Blake and Freddie Feltham. You know how much you mean to me. Lastly, thank you to Humphrey Heylen, for everything.

El Blackwood
2024

Tending was first performed on 1st August 2024 at Underbelly Cowgate as part of the Edinburgh Fringe Festival.

CAST

NURSE 1:	**Ben Lynn**
NURSE 2:	**El Blackwood**
NURSE 3:	**Mara Allen**

CREATIVES

Writer:	**El Blackwood**
Director & Dramaturg:	**John Livesey**
Producer:	**Eleanor Birdsall-Smith**

ABOUT THE CAST AND CREATIVES

Ben Lynn | Actor *(Nurse 1)*

Ben Lynn trained at RADA. Theatre credits include: *As You Like It* (Lord Chamberlain's Men); *The Malcontent, Dido Queen of Carthage* (Shakespeare's Globe), *Monster, Red Velvet, Against, Kursk* (RADA).

Film credits include *Ghostbusters—Frozen Empire*.

Ben also completed a foundation course at The Cambridge School of Visual and Performing Arts.

El Blackwood | Writer & Actor *(Nurse 2)*

El Blackwood is an actor, writer and producer. El trained as a playwright on the prestigious John Burgess Playwriting Course (2021-2022) and as an actor with Identity School of Acting (2021-2023) and the Orange Tree Theatre Young Company (2022-2023). El is also the co-founder of Offshoots Theatre, which platforms and connects emerging creatives while raising money for the Trussell Trust. In 2023, she founded El Blackwood Productions and wrote the award-winning play, *Tending*. *Tending* achieved critical and commercial success at Edinburgh Fringe 2023, and was invited back for a month-long run at Underbelly in 2024. Lastly, El was selected as one of eight playwrights to be a Brixton House 'housemate', winning a funded week-long run in October 2024.

Mara Allen | Actor *(Nurse 3)*

Mara graduated from The Royal Academy of Dramatic Arts (RADA) in 2019. Theatre credits include: *The Night Watch* (The Original Theatre Company), *Macbeth (*The Globe Theatre, Playing Shakespeare with Deutsche Bank), *Henry V* (OVO production at The Maltings Theatre), *A Midsummer Night's Dream* (The Changeling Theatre Company), *Jacaranda* (The Pentabus Theatre Company), *An Octoroon* (The Abbey Theatre, Dublin), *The Mirror Crack'd* (The Original Theatre Company) and *King Lear* (The Kenneth Branagh Theatre Company).

TV/Film credits including: *Romantic Getaway* (SKY Comedy).

John Livesey | Director & Dramaturg

John Livesey is a writer, dramaturg and director. He has directed multiple shows including *random* (Actor's Centre, 2020), *Heather* (Southwark Playhouse, 2021), and *Amphibian* (King's Head Theatre, Hannah Barry Gallery; 2022). John trained on the Stone Crabs Young Directors Programme and with OUDS, the Oxford University Drama Society. For his work on *random*, he was selected to take part in the National Student Drama Festival. John is a member of The North Wall Arts Lab programme and, in 2023, was selected for the Independent Film Trust's Talent Led programme and the Punchdrunk Young Talent Network. In 2024, he was selected by the European Theatre Convention to take part in an artist residency at the Deutsches Theater, Berlin. He is working on a PhD with University College London, and is the recipient of an AHRC research scholarship.

Eleanor Birdsall-Smith | Producer

Eleanor Birdsall-Smith is a producer and freelancer. She has worked in Film and TV production, including on projects for Netflix, HBO and Sony, and is a former junior agent at Independent Talent. Eleanor produced the recent sold-out run of *Cowboys and Lesbians* at Park Theatre as well as its Fringe run and first iteration as *Scholar's Creek* in January 2022, which secured full Arts Council funding. She also produces for screen, including a number of acclaimed music videos for the band *Pynch* and the upcoming short film *Fair Weather.*

v

CHARACTERS

NURSE 1

Male, 25—35. Palliative care nurse. Professional, gentle, supportive of patients and his peers.

NURSE 2

Female/NB, 25—35. Paediatric ICU nurse. Highly empathetic, heart-on-her-sleeve type. Very popular with parents. Often becomes overly involved with her patients.

NURSE 3

Female/NB, 25—45. A&E nurse. Boundaried, highly practical, a 'doer'. Occasionally sarcastic. Moralistic.

NB:

All three nurses were transferred to Adult ICU during three waves of Covid.

NOTE ON COSTUME

Following hospital rules, nails must not be painted. Any items worn under scrubs must be considered through the lens of infection control. Long hair should be tied back.

This script represents the play at the time of rehearsal and there could be changes during the production.

SCENE 1

Blackout.

Projected text appears. It states "Tending is based on 70 interviews with NHS nurses."

Then, "Everything you hear on stage today has been said by a nurse."

Blackout.

A voice clip plays of a woman speaking candidly about her decision to become a nurse. Then another voice clip, this time a man. Then another. And another. Slowly these excerpts build and build, creating a choir, and then a cacophony of voices. The volume continues to increase. Until...

Silence.

Lights up.

Three figures appear upstage, standing in front of three chairs. All wear scrub trousers and plain t-shirts. Each considers the space in front of them downstage, as if looking at a microphone. They look at us. All of them have different, changing facial expressions: each feeling differently about the prospect of speaking.

NURSE 1 approaches the front of the stage.

NURSE 1: Umm.

NURSE 3 strides to the front of the stage.

NURSE 3: What's this for again?

NURSE 2 tentatively approaches the front of the stage. She hesitates.

We hear a strange, watery, rumble. She is embarrassed.

NURSE 2: Sorry, that was my stomach.

Beat.

NURSE 1: So this is for a play?

NURSE 3: So this is for a play?

NURSE 2: So this is for a play?

Pause.

Well, you were like, have you ever thought about nursing?

Beat.

And I actually hadn't at all.

NURSE 3: I was actually dead set against nursing.
My mum's a nurse as well and I didn't wanna be like my mum.
That's what you're like when you're a teenager.

NURSE 1: (*chuckles*) I was a medicine convert. I didn't get the grades to do medicine. Got a job as a Healthcare Assistant.

NURSE 3: I remember thinking: I wanna be a PE teacher, I'm gonna do work experience in that. I went in to do work experience. Hated it, obviously.

NURSE 1: It was chatting to the nurses on the trauma ward I worked on. Just talking to them. I realised everything that I wanted to get out of medicine I could eventually get from nursing.

NURSE 2: I remember watching a video of these neonatal intensive care nurses in a warzone.
And this hospital had just been hit and was slowly crumbling. Watching them strapping these babies to themselves and just running. I just couldn't comprehend the human capacity to go so far.
So that got me thinking.

NURSE 3: Just down by my school there was a hospital, like a rehab hospital for brain injuries? I went and spent a week with them, I was sixteen/seventeen? I guess that's when I kind of realised.

2

NURSE 2: I was like maybe I'll do children's nursing cuz I like kids. They scare me a bit, but I like kids. And then what I thought nursing was... rapidly changed.

NURSE 3: You kind of just fall more in love with your job, as tough as it can be sometimes. Now I'm a band 6 in A&E. I'm also trained in ICU... so a bit of everything.

NURSE 1: There's a lack of, um, sort of personal connection that I found from most of the doctors that I came across. And I saw the relationships that nurses had with patients, relatives, carers and things...
Patients don't care if they get their drugs on time, if their observations are alright. They care if you know how they like their cup of tea. Do you know what I mean?
I think I just thought I'd get more satisfaction from that.

NURSE 2: It's like, you know, helping people. And... like being seen as someone that's capable of anything. It's the first time you're given the responsibility of another human being's life and it's on you.

SCENE 2

Three people are on stage, carrying out their morning routine. NURSE 1 eats cereal —sloppily, NURSE 2 brushes their teeth with headphones in—bopping, NURSE 3 does their makeup in a rush.

Blackout. They are gone.

We hear the sound of tube doors closing. Then the sound of hospital doors opening. The lights brighten and the sounds of a busy ward surround the space. These sounds continue at a low-level. It's the beginning of the working day.

NURSE 2: So, arrive at work. I start at 7.30.

NURSE 3 and NURSE 1 turn and move upstage to pull on their scrubs whilst NURSE 2 describes her routine.

Sometimes you're rushing, sometimes you're on time.
Get changed into your scrubs. You're not allowed to wear
uniform on public transport because of infection control.
Anxiety kicks in.

NURSE 3: Before you even walk onto the ward. You can kind of
work out what your day is going to look like. Just by seeing
the body language of the other nurses on shift.

The nurses notice each other for the first time. NURSE 2 puts on their scrub top.

NURSE 1: Are they relaxed, chatting?

NURSE 2: Or are people rushing around like there's still things
left to be done?

NURSE 3: You sit in hand over. Like a coffee room, basically.
There's like 50 nurses in there.

NURSE 2: You get a quick handover of like, the patients on the
ward, and then you get sent Out. It smells like cleaning fluid.

NURSE 2: For intensive care you do all of your safety checks,
figure out what meds are needed and when.
If they need to have any X-ray scans: see any specialists, speak
with family, update on plans, speak with doctor, plans, lots of
plans and tasks.

NURSE 3: Monotonous drug round, observations after that, then
the doctors come round with all the tasks that need done: any
bloods, ECGs, catheters, (*pfft*) lunchtime medications.

NURSE 2: Poo, poo, poo. Wee, wee, wee. Sick. Blood. Secretions.
All through the day. Constant.

NURSE 3: More drugs. it's never the same.

NURSE 2: And you're constantly helping other nurses. Intensive
care especially is amazing teamwork, cos you can't do it
without each other.

NURSE 2 begins to mime turning a great weight.

You can't turn a full-sized adult by yourself.

The two nurses step in, the weight becomes manageable and they move in motion easily.

And that's an amazing thing.
The teamwork, when it's fluid, it's/

NURSE 2: /effortless.

NURSE 2 returns upstage. They conduct routine movements, like hanging up a fluid bag and putting on a fob watch.

NURSE 3: In A&E, right at the start, we're not that busy.
Probably by 11 o'clock, people are queuing out the door to come in and it just gets busier and busier from then on.
And you've got to take into account that an emergency can be wheeled through those doors at any time.

NURSE 1: Er, I probably triage—see—three hundred odd people a day? Maybe more, the bank holiday was particularly bad.
You try and get a break. Hopefully a bit of breakfast and then a lunch break anytime between 1 and 6pm, depending on the day, how well-staffed you are.

NURSE 2 faces the audience, scrub top now on, as if they were a mirror. As the other nurses speak, she does her hair, pulls at the hem of her shirt, and takes deep breaths.

NURSE 3: I haven't come across much material that's very realistic of what it's like to be a nurse, now. Lots of postwar *(laughing)*... what's that show called?

NURSES 1 & 2: Call the midwife!

NURSE 3: I probably drink about 200ml of fluid a day. If I'm lucky I might get a coffee to keep me going. And then on my days off I'll make up for it so that I don't get a UTI.

NURSE 1: I feel like a normal job would allow us to have like one sandwich?

NURSE 3: And maybe a pee break?

NURSE 2 joins them downstage.

We wash the patients as well.
When I'm washing someone who is sedated I'm always like,
speaking and asking consent and telling them what I'm doing.

NURSE 2: I think my most important thing is that like I never
want anyone to feel shame. Because like, I know what that
feels like.

NURSE 3: I just do a really good job. I'm a clean ***bitch***. I would
also want to be a clean person. Like if I'm gonna wash you, I'm
gonna wash you well.

NURSE 2: Am I allowed to talk about poo?

The nurses look at each other, as if daring each other to speak first.

NURSE 1: I think you'd be lying if you said you enjoyed wiping
bums.

NURSE 3: When the memory of a smell, the memory of a smell
makes you gag, you know it's bad.

NURSE 2: Yeah.

NURSE 3: It's so hard to describe smells accurately.

NURSE 2: No it was so bad. It was like burning evil.

They're making each other laugh.

NURSE 1: Literally it feels like it's burning. That's how bad
smells can get.

NURSE 3: Yeah.

NURSE 2: Like do you remember when the ventilation broke?

NURSE 3: Oh, this is a story/

NURSE 2: /and we were getting the leftover smell from the
kidney dialysis unit pumped into ours?

NURSE 1: And they wouldn't close the unit or do anything about it.

NURSE 2: There's definitely been times where I've been like, I'm gonna be sick in my mouth.

NURSE 1: Yeah.

NURSE 2: Like the amount of times we've been cleaning, or turning someone and they start farting.

NURSE 1: And I make eye contact with you, and you're just like no, no, no, no, no.

NURSE 2: Just like this lava descends from a bottle and you're looking at each other. And you kind of freeze. You're just like, it's happening now. I'll just let it happen.

NURSE 3: And a lot of intensive care patients, they're so constipated from all the drugs. That when they finally go, it's like, thank God, but my God is this Satanic.

NURSE 2: There was one that made me cry. It was so pungent like/

NURSE 1: /The antibiotics make it really stunning as well.

NURSE 2: Yeah. Really like, like, like really sharp in the nose.

NURSE 3: You think poo is just like a poo smell, but poo can be worse. Poo can be like, poo squared.

The lighting suddenly changes. The room turns cold, and NURSE 2 seems to want to say something.

She steps forward.

NURSE 2: There was this girl, 15.

She stops. She takes a deep breath and starts again.

There was this girl, 15. And she was very tall, like very tall.

SCENE 3

The Lighting changes abruptly. The warmth returns to the room and NURSE 2 takes a step back. For a minute she hesitates, and then returns to the moment.

NURSE 1: The night shift is definitely more relaxed.

NURSE 3: Sometimes we put like, Smooth Radio on, really quietly? Just to blackout the noise a bit from outside.

NURSE 1: We have like three or four machines attached to every patient and every single one has a different alarm.

NURSE 2: All different types of beeps and levels of beeps.

NURSE 3: If one certain sound on a ventilator stops happening, the ventilation has stopped.

NURSE 2: The machines have got like different squeaks to them. And if the squeak stops, you hear the squeak stopping before the alarm starts.

NURSE 1: And so everybody clicks on to that sound and everyone goes,

ALL: Is that machine going?!

NURSE 3: I swear to God, I've gone home after shifts, and I've genuinely heard these noises in my sleep and thought I'm still at work.

NURSE 1: You'll just go home and hear beep, beep, beep.

NURSE 2: In the NICU, there's so much soothing white noise, for the babies. Just like shh shh shh shh shh just like that rhythm. And the pat pats.

NNURSE 2 pats her chest rhythmically.

That soothing, steady kind of beat. Shh shh shh shh shh.

NURSE 1: We try and encourage minimal handling. Minimum involvement.

NURSE 2: We try to turn the lights down, if the patient's not very sick.

NURSE 3: We get a lot of dementia patients who are confused and need someone to sit with them at night and just stroking them there...
Until they'd fall asleep.

NURSE 1: I remember I used to spend nights talking to this guy. I'm not gonna say his name obviously but like, every time I was on a night shift we would talk all night and he would tell me all of the things he'd like to do when he gets better.

NURSE 2: It's always freezing, I don't know why.

NURSE 3: Everyone's cold on a night shift.

NURSE 2: There are all these hospital trolleys that have mattresses on. Don't tell anyone but sometimes...

NURSE 2 goes to her chair upstage, and drags it downstage.

Sometimes I drag a mattress off the trolley into the staff toilets, whack a sheet down and (*wistfully*) set an alarm for twenty minutes.

She collapses into the chair.

NURSE 3: And when that alarm goes off, and you're like...

ALL: Urghhhh!

NURSE 3: That's pretty devastating.

NURSE 3 collapses into her chair.

NURSE 2: Sometimes I would literally sleep in a cupboard, on the floor. Like I'd lay down a towel and just like, just like fold up. I was so tired.

NURSE 3: It's like a little secret that goes on in the nursing world. Everyone knows that everyone does it, but it's not official.

NURSE 1: You'll just see a Healthcare Assistant sat in a chair, fast asleep.

NURSE 3: I love doing a Saturday night though. The amount of people who come in drunk is actually just funny. Drunk patients who do not need to be there.

NURSE 1 goes to say something, demandingly. Nurse 3 holds a hand up.

If you're well enough to argue with me, you're well enough to go home!

NURSE 1: I know all of us in ED whenever we finish our last night shift we all get a McDonalds breakfast, because I think it's a must.

SCENE 4

NURSE 3: My best memory?

NURSE 2: I really, really enjoy getting patients off the ventilator. It's actually waking them up, getting them into their parents' arms, letting them have a cuddle for the first time.

NURSE 3: When the kids would be well enough to experience joy.

NURSE 1: If they've been attached to medications and not been able to leave the bedspace, then get a little bit better, we get a portable stand and a wheelchair, and just fly them around the unit.

They run with a chair, joyously.

NURSE 2: It's hard for parents to be there all the time, especially if they've got other kids. So I'm kind of a surrogate parent... surrogate mum/

NURSE 1: /Another beautiful memory I have is with patients, like when they come back and hug you and tell you 'I wouldn't have made it without you'.

NURSE 2: And you know you're gonna miss them, and you know, maybe something will happen but in that moment they're good.

NURSE 1: It's being able to take people outside for the first time. Cause we've got a helipad now at the hospital and it's... you know it's up on the 11th floor and you get views all over London.
It's seeing people's faces when they get to see that.

Beat.

NURSE 1: The other thing that pops into my mind is the bed round.

NURSE 2: Ooh, doing the beds with my colleagues.

NURSE 3: Someone would say something like horrendously funny. Because you're working with some seriously funny people, who could always make you laugh. And I think I was that to some people too.

NURSE 1: Cat walking down the corridor with like a poo in a komode, like fucking voguing/

NURSE 2: /and like putting on music/

NURSE 1: /And I know cos you're in a hospital, you have to be professional. But when I was allowed to be by myself with my colleagues and my patients that was my favourite.

NURSE 2: Every Friday morning, before we start work, we choose a song and dance to it.

Music blares. 15 seconds of Titanium by Sia plays. They perform a coordinated routine that disintegrates into freestyling. They are joyous. The music cuts. They stop dancing.

SCENE 5

The lighting is soft, warm and inviting. There is a calmness in the soundscape.

NURSE 1: Small acts of care... um, tea. Tea for parents, tea for patients.

NURSE 3: Food, feeding people.

NURSE 2: Picking out outfits for them.

NURSE 1: Brushing hair.

NURSE 3: Washing hair.

NURSE 2: There was this amazing nurse in children's intensive care. Have I told you about him? We called him John Frieda because he'd... there was like this extension you can add to the bed where you can wash patients' hair when they were in a medical coma. And he'd wash their hair, and plait it so beautifully.

NURSE 3: It's rare. It's rare in the NHS, those moments. It's like, stretched so thin.

NURSE 1: It is the little things, I think. Like compression socks? I always pull the toe bits so the toes aren't squished.

NURSE 2: Hand massages, to calm patients down.

NURSE 3: Buying things I know they'd like on my break.

NURSE 1: A six pack of cold coke.

NURSE 3: Chocolate.

NURSE 2: Stickers. I spent all my student loan on stickers.

NURSE 3: I am a very tactile person. So I am not frightened to just put my arm around patients or hold their hand.

NURSE 1: I had a patient who was a vicar, on Christmas Eve, so I played hymns for him all night. And every time I was like... are the hymns annoying you? He'd just shake his head, to keep playing them.

NURSE 2: There was this young guy, late 20s. Late-stage cancer. He had loads of mouth sores. See, oncology drugs often give you awful adhesions. And you have these lollipop sticks, they're pink sponges on white sticks, and you dip them in water and press them onto lips to stop them drying out. And it was kind of Christ-like, you know, this young guy, sitting in bed... dying, and I'm pressing this sponge of water to his mouth.
He was just saying this is, this is heavenly. This has been so sore, and that's really helping me. He could barely speak. I think he died 10 days later. But I've never forgotten him.

A pause.

NURSE 2 and NURSE 3 fold a sheet, move objects, adjust the room unaware. NURSE 1 remains still, and focused on the audience.

NURSE 1: There's so many different types of nursing, and I've only experienced a slither of it, but it is... love. Nursing when it's good is love. It's loving strangers. Because you're trying to heal someone. And like clinical excellence is so important. But there are so many things, that aren't that, with nursing that keep people alive. And I had no idea what that meant. Until I started.

SCENE 6

NURSE 3: The love of the profession is so there for people that are a part of it. But/

NURSE 1 & NURSE 2: The paperwork.

NURSE 3: When you're training, they drum into you...

NURSE 1 becomes the overbearing trainer, as NURSE 2 and NURSE 3 run around, trying to carry out tasks.

NURSE 1: "If you haven't documented that, you haven't done it."

NURSE 2 and NURSE 3 sigh.

NURSE 3: I don't mind the little tick boxes, we have for like your catheter and your cannula—it's having to write up every little thing/

NURSE 1: /I almost felt like I was more like a secretary. I was doing more paperwork than I was actually doing hands on, one to one, with... with my patients.

NURSE 2: 80 per cent of my day was spent doing paperwork and 20 per cent was left to look after the patients and I think it should be the other way around.

All three NURSES mime air quotation marks.

NURSE 3: "The patient is a client." You just do your job, you're done.

NURSE 1: But when you're there, it's not that simple.

They begin to fold paper planes, differing in their levels of intricacy.

NURSE 3: For me personally, I'm a little bit stubborn, so I would just end up spending an hour sitting on a chair with a patient talking to them and not give a shit about my paperwork.

NURSE 2: What paperwork creates, it creates one person who is accountable for one mistake, and that one person has to pay for it.

NURSE 1: And you're like, I'm looking after eleven people, by myself of course there's going to be a mistake? The numbers don't match, and then you give me all of these things I should be... writing about?

NURSE 3: It's all about money and budgets. And that's not what nursing's about, nursing's about human beings.

They throw their paper planes.

NURSE 2: There was this girl, 15.

She stops. She takes a deep breath and starts again.

There was this girl, 15. And she was very tall, like very tall. I remember she took up the whole bed.

SCENE 7

NURSE 1: I'm quite passionate about palliative care. End of life care.

NURSE 3: There's a sort of slogan that is like 'one chance to get it right'.

NURSE 1: I find it such a privilege, you know, caring for someone at the end of their life. It's like being at someone's birth.

NURSE 2: It's, it's exactly the same. You do it once. That's it. That's all they're gonna have and witness.

NURSE 1: We've got people's dogs to come in, snuck them onto the unit so that they could say goodbye to their dog.
The hospital across the water they got someone's horse. It's quite grassy. So the patient could say goodbye to that horse.

NURSE 3: When I worked in a hospice, we had a budgie in once. Belonged to this woman. And then she died and they got stuck with the budgie for like two years? It used to freak them out because it used to go dead quiet when people were dying. It wouldn't sing.

NURSE 1: There's been weddings. There've been quite a lot of weddings.
There's a facebook page where sometimes, um, one of the wards will put like 'Planning a last-minute wedding. Does anyone know anyone that could do flowers, a cake, that sort of thing?'

Pause.

NURSE 3: In the hospital, you kinda see the guts of life a bit, you know what I mean?

NURSE 2: Yeah. People are vulnerable, are suffering. You're close up to like, the human condition or whatever you want to call it.

NURSE 1: And seeing that, in my mind, makes it easier to understand stuff. One day we are all going to get sick, we are all going to die.

NURSE 3: I remember there was this one person she was 28 or 29 and she was so nice, six months' pregnant.

She was so excited about this pregnancy, she was like knitting stuff for the baby. She arrived and we were just talking a lot and then during the procedure we found out that she had this massive tumour.

It was just in a position where she couldn't... she had to interrupt the pregnancy to remove the tumour. She had to be operated on the next week. I had to go there and tell her that she had to get rid of the baby or she would die and the baby too.

And it's like... how do you tell her that?

Everytime things like that happen I'm like what if this was me? What if it was my sister? What if it was my mum? Every time.

Pause.

NURSE 1: In December I was on a run of four nights. On the second night, it was rainy and dark, and there was a trauma call. He'd been on a Christmas night out in a bar in town. He'd slipped down some stairs and cracked his head open.

We got him in, tried to work out what we could do with him. The answer was not a lot. It was a catastrophic brain bleed. He was only 40.

His wife arrived, um, and she was lovely. He had a thirteen-year-old and a fifteen-year-old daughter as well. And then I ended up getting invited to his funeral. It's the first, and probably only patient funeral I'll ever go to.

I learnt a lot about him and his life. Then, at the end of his eulogy, they mentioned me by name.

By that point I was absolutely sobbing because... I had two days in that 40-year-old man's life. And that was one of the things that the family felt was important. I knew him for 48 hours if that?

NURSE 2: Some kids need a tracheostomy, which is like a little hole in your windpipe and a little tube allows them to breathe. The thing about having a trachy is that they can have a speaking valve but otherwise it takes your voice away.

There was this kid, when he'd laugh it was silent but his whole face would squish up and his eyes would go so small and he looked like The Incredibles baby?

And his mum was amazing, 19, and just fearless. And I always said to her you'd be a brilliant nurse, and she always said no no no, only for him. Only for him.

NURSE 3: A lot of the time people outside healthcare think that the parents don't want to speak about the happy times, but they do. Or what school they went to or their favourite subject. We do like clay hand prints, foot prints. A lock of hair, playing music, playing their favourite show.

NURSE 2: When you've looked after someone so long, every day, it's very easy to forget that he's probably not going to live past four if he's lucky, but like... I'll do what I can to give him a very full life in that time.

There were moments where I'd care for him and it was like, pure joy, watching him reach milestones where he could somewhat sit up and moments of pure terror, where he'd go a bit blue, and I'd have to shout for help, and I'd have to give him the breaths.

We all loved him a lot.

And then one day, a week from going home, something just went wrong. And like, no one could save him. And he just died.

The heartbeat stops.

For a moment, silence.

I read it in an email. I guess they do that so you can digest it in your own time and space.

Slowly, the sound of a hospital starts to build.

NURSE 3: When you're newly qualified you don't have... you have no idea.
It's like learning to drive isn't it? The minute that your L-plates come off, it's very different.
Erm, and you have to learn everything over again. And I remember the charge, literally the first thing he said to me was:

NURSE 1: "You'll all cry for the first six months of your career, every day."

NURSE 3: And we all didn't believe him, but it was bang on. It was true. Erm, and then six months later/

NURSE 2: /Covid hit.

SCENE 8

All three nurses are upstage. News excerpts from 2020 play, the UK is in Lockdown. Each remembers. The sounds build. They begin to walk slowly forward.

NURSE 2: I remember the first time/

NURSE 3: /That first shift.

NURSE 1: We'd spent like 15 minutes donning PPE. And then the doors opened.

NURSE 2: It just looked futuristic. It looked like you were walking onto a spaceship.

NURSE 1: I'd seen the news clips about what had gone on, and then the doors opened and I actually walked into it.

NURSE 3: Those first, that first month was terrifying.

NURSE 2: Beeping, lots of beeping, you've got the heart rate monitors

Sounds mirror her words.

You've got the oxygen saturations, you've got the IV pumps. You've got like blood machines running, ventilator sounds, alarms.
So many alarms going off constantly. Someone shouting for help. Another person shouting for help.

NURSE 1: "Where are you?"

NURSE 3: I was like screaming down the walkie-talkie, like frantically like...

NURSE 1: "Where are you?" And they're like...

NURSE 3: "We're just putting on our PPE!"

NURSE 2: Patients like calling out and no one coming to them because no one's available, because someone's stopped breathing and everyone is there.

NURSE 1: And then another person stops breathing and you've got to do CPR.

NURSE 3: I'm waiting for people to come in like this is horrendous. And then you'd work with amazing seniors that would just say fuck PPE, walk straight in. 'Cause they knew what it was. It was a matter of seconds.

NURSE 1: Getting home, being like, not gonna speak to my Mum. It was like straight in, upstairs, clothes into a bag, shower. Wouldn't stay in the same room cuz she's at risk.

NURSE 2: Someone's pulled their tube out because they're under-sedated, another emergency. Phone's ringing. Someone's playing a radio somewhere.

NURSE 1: Watching so many people die and not being able to stop it.

NURSE 2: Someone's laughing about something.

NURSE 3: People just say do your best, but when that's someone's life, it just doesn't really cut it?

NURSE 2: Patients screaming, crying, phone's ringing, alarms going. Whispering. Laughing. Crying. Screaming. All of it. Every sound you can imagine.

Beat.

Sorry, can I just take a moment?

Sounds stop.

NURSE 3: Where do you feel it in your body, when you think about those sounds?

NURSE 2: My chest, definitely. Just like a huge pressure.

NURSE 1: Here?

NURSE 2: Yeah. On my chest.

NURSE 1: Like someone sitting on your chest.

Beat.

SCENE 9

NURSE 2: I think back to stuff that I did at the start of Covid and I was like, oh, I missed that. I didn't know that. Like I wonder if I'd done that differently, whether or not, you know, they wouldn't have deteriorated.

NURSE 3: You couldn't help but feel like that was your fault.

NURSE 2: One of my patients, he was mid to late 70s, and he was a new admission. He was really scared, really scared. He was getting really sick. And he kept taking his mask off. It got to a point where I was pleading with him.

NURSE 1: You need to keep this on, like you have to keep this on, you can't breathe without it.

NURSE 2: He was on Facetime with his daughters. And they were like...

NURSE 3: Please, if we could just come see him, we can calm him down.

NURSE 2: They were begging me. I said I'm sorry, I'm sorry. I can't let you in, that's not within my power. And they were, you know. And it was just so heartbreaking because if that was my Dad like, fuck you telling me not to come in. No doubt it would have calmed him down.
And then the next day I came in and he was intubated, and then he died that night.
It was just so quick.
And like, I knew. I knew he was going to die and that's such a crazy thing to know? To look at someone and think, you're gonna die. Yeah I just couldn't stop thinking about my Dad.

NURSE 1: My Dad was constantly like, just quit. Just quit. I was like, I have two months' notice. He was like, you can take it off. Just quit. I don't care. Like immediately come home. And I was like, I just can't. Like, you just can't, like people die. I just can't.
I can still hear the voicenotes that family would send in. We'd put them on the pillow and we'd play them. Things like "oh we're painting the gate for when you get home", and they'd die the next day.

NURSE 2: I personally, I personally like bagged up 40 people, maybe 50 people. We cleared the wards that I was on, which was 25-bed ward, four times. When we ran out of bags, we wrapped them in sheets and stuff like what we could find. It's just like, this isn't dignified. This isn't nice.

NURSE 3: I just remember both my sisters crying when they saw me. And I was like, shit, man, this is bad.
All my hair started snapping off. And I had like an allergic

reaction to a face mask. So I had like this red like, uh, raw, flaky skin around my face.

NURSE 2: I know some people have got physical scars on their face, from the PPE.

NURSE 3: And then like obviously I was really just dehydrated the entire time. So like really sunken eyes and it looked terrible. Yeah, I remember they just started crying they were like, I can't believe they're doing this to you. And I was like, I have no choice.
Those shifts, like I just couldn't even lift my head off the sofa, some days I was so exhausted.

NURSE 1: Normally, I like really try to steady my hands. I dunno if you've noticed. I'm like... my hands have to be steady. But my hands got so shaky.

NURSE 3: I went home and I slept. I slept so hard with no dreams.

NURSE 2: It was just like no time. Like living in pockets of adrenaline constantly.

NURSE 1: At that point I knew...

NURSE 3: I've lost too much of myself.

NURSE 1: I can't keep giving what I'm giving.

The lighting suddenly changes. The room turns cold, and NURSE 2 seems to want to say something.

NURSE 2: There was this girl, 15.

She stops. She takes a deep breath and starts again.

There was this girl, 15. And she was very tall, like very tall. She had this fiery red hair. She wasn't my patient. But she came on my shift, so I...

NURSE 2 falters.

SCENE 10

The lighting changes to neutral.

NURSE 3: I think it can actually be quite a lonely life, to be a nurse. I come home and I don't wanna talk and I don't wanna do things. I just want to be mute.

NURSE 1: I remember I stopped even just saying things out loud when I got home. You're expected to be so strong and so resilient.

NURSE 3: And then you come home and the people around you want you to be the same thing for them and you think I want someone to take care of me?

NURSE 2: My heart is like a balloon, like by the end of the day it's just empty. I just want to go on TikTok and dissociate.

NURSE 1: You have to dissociate. Cuz if you took everything home, you probably wouldn't have a career.

NURSE 3: They always chuck around this word 'resilience' and I hate that word.

NURSE 2: Everyone's like, oh, 'we need to build up resilience'. You need to build resilience to this and that. And it's like, we're going through things that are sort of unheard of.

NURSE 1: This illusion that nurses are kind of unbreakable/

NURSE 2: /behind every nurse is a whole spiderweb of life that is going on and affecting their ability to nurse, essentially.

NURSE 3: I woke up one night. And I just felt like I was gonna be sick. I couldn't eat. There was this dread, which wasn't new. I'd felt that throughout the whole pandemic. And a lot of my job. That dread feeling when you're so tired.
But I was like... gotta go. And I got in my car. And then... started driving. And it was like, weirdly bad traffic.
I was like half way through, it was just before that huge

roundabout at Elephant and Castle I cant remember what that road is called. And I just I just froze?

And people started beeping, but I think I dissociated for like a minute. And when I came to I was like fuck. I indicated and pulled over.

But it was very calm. It was like my body was like 'this is not for negotiation.' You're not going any further.

So I called my nurse in charge. She picked up, and was like...

NURSE 1: Hello?

NURSE 3: She sounded exhausted herself. And I told her I just I can't.

NURSE 1: What do you mean?

NURSE 3: I can't... I can't do this.

Pause.

She just knew. She was like...

NURSE 1: OK, go home. If you can't do it you can't do it.

NURSE 3: Um, and then it was like... I don't know at that point I knew that was it for me.

And then I just cried, continuously for 72 hours.

Until I was dry. I felt such a mixture of things. Shame and just like heartbreak for all of my friends that had to go and do it and they'd be a nurse down. What that would mean for them? When I spoke to my GP it was amazing. I didn't really need to say anything. She just said what's the reason for calling? And I said, Oh, I'm a nurse working in ICU and she said OK, I've signed you off for two months. Is that enough? I was like Oh, I don't, I don't know.

NURSE 1: I think they only came around with access to like psychologists and things like that sort of halfway through Covid? One of the nurses committed suicide in the hospital.

NURSE 3: This is the new norm. This is what we're expected to do. And this is not gonna change anytime soon.

NURSE 2: And feeling, feeling the impact of that. There are so many of us that if one of us falls, who cares?

The lighting suddenly changes. The room turns cold, and NURSE 2 seems to want to say something.

NURSE 2: I remember she took up the whole bed. She had this fiery red hair, like mine.

She stops. She takes a deep breath and tries again.

I felt very conflicted.
She had been on day release from this like, assisted living for people that were suffering quite severely from mental health issues.
I just remember being like (*deep breath*) I dunno if we've done the right thing.

SCENE 11

NURSE 1 and NURSE 2 busy themselves. They perform routine tasks quickly. NURSE 3 seems distant from them.

NURSE 3: You can see stress.

NURSE 3 watches them.

You try and learn to deal with it.

NURSE 1: If I'm still on the ward, I go to the bathroom because it's the only place I can be alone.

NURSE 3: I think I've always felt things so intensely. It's annoying.

NURSE 2: I get in my car and put on a song. I sit, and cry, and sing.

NURSE 1: Sit down, take a minute.

NURSE 2: It's little things.

NURSE 3: I think we forget touch is really important.

NURSE 1: If I see a colleague who's stressed.

NURSE 1 approaches NURSE 2

I place my hand on their back, and you feel them sort of melt?

NURSE 2 relaxes into their hand.

NURSE 3: Hugs. So many hugs that other nurses have given me.

NURSE 2: And then ones I've been like, don't. Don't do that. Because I'll lose it. Or so many times where I'll be like no! No! Don't be nice to me. You know? Cos it's like, I'll break.

SCENE 12

NURSE 3: We had the Health Minister come in when I was on shift, and they wouldn't let him speak to any of the nurses on the floor.

NURSE 2: They just try and make it look like we're coping absolutely fine? Because they don't want to say we're not?

NURSE 1: We had an MP who came in as a patient.

NURSE 3: There's a whole policy and protocol.

NURSE 1: As soon as they booked in they got a bed, ridiculously early, whereas most of the time people are sat in chairs for fifty hours.

NURSE 3: The people that are managing the hospitals and running the whole health service, you know: they don't know. They wander through the department saying, well why hasn't that patient had this? Because the nurse is dealing with another sick patient, and I haven't got another nurse to do it.

NURSE 2: They don't come to the people on the floor to ask them. What do you need?

NURSE 1: There's no staff support, the only time they listen is when a patient complains and even then... it's just demoralising because we work so hard and we try our best but our best is not good enough, and it's just...

NURSE 2: When things happen, nothing changes.

NURSE 3: I remember when a mental health patient locked himself in the toilet, in A&E. The toilets don't have a lock from the outside. By the time that we'd managed to get the door off he'd smashed the sink up and as soon as we opened the door he slit his throat in front of me.
And he did a good job, he didn't hit the carotid, but he hit the jugular. So straight away my arm went into his neck and he went straight to theater.
But then, that would be a lesson to say "We need to change the doors on that, we need a safer environment."
Has anything changed? No. The door is still... you can't unlock it from the outside.

NURSE 2: The most painful bit for me is that like Everyone just keeps going/

NURSE 1: /You're doing three people's jobs most of the time, maybe even more, and then you're taking on so much work that you just, keep going somehow, until you physically can't/

NURSE 3: For a caring profession, it's very uncaring to its workers, I think.

NURSE 2: I just remember sometimes feeling like screaming, being like, until you are in it, you really don't know the weight of what we're carrying. Without any support.

NURSE 3: A lot of sick days, a lot of leave, a lot of, like, I saw people break down, um, you know, break down in tears and not be able to cope.

NURSE 2: Or the opposite, which was to become so robotic in their nature, as if nothing could touch them.

NURSE 1: I was like a robot. It feels horrible saying this but when I wasn't on a unit, I could just walk down... I could walk down a corridor of patients and look down constantly because I didn't want to make eye contact because I didn't have time to help them. And it'd just stay like that for twelve hours. It was just... so dehumanising/

NURSE 2: People get burnt out and think "I just can't do this anymore" you know I just cannot do this anymore... and then you get compassion fatigue and that is the worst possible thing you can have when you're trying to look after people.

NURSE 3: I'm a patient person. I've always prided myself on that and all of a sudden I just realised I'm not, I'm not patient anymore.

NURSE 1: You can't turn up to the shift and give the amount of empathy, care, compassion.

NURSE 2: And then we had this massive issue of like, the best, the people who know the place inside out, who know the patients, and are basically like the pillars of the place leaving/

NURSE 1: /because they've been forced out.

SCENE 13

Sound clips play of the 2023 nurses strikes.

NURSE 1: It was so loud. I don't think the clips on the news got across how loud it was.

NURSE 2: People on megaphones.

NURSE 3: The amount of people who were there just shouting, chanting.

NURSE 2: And the cars, buses and lorries, beeping as they went past.

NURSE 3: When ambulances and police cars went past they put on their sirens, everyone was going past honking.

NURSE 1: We did have one woman drive past with her thumbs down like that...

NURSE 3 mimes the outraged woman, she makes the others laugh.

but there weren't really any people against it. Everyone was supporting it/

NURSE 2: /People dropping off food, people dropping off cakes, most importantly people dropping off hot drinks.

NURSE 1: It was fucking cold because it was December.

NURSE 2: So everyone was all sort of wrapped up and like huddled together.

NURSE 3: I had a hot water bottle in my coat and a hot water bottle on my feet.

NURSE 2: Someone gave me gloves. A builder I think he was giving me like those thick gloves builders use because my hands were bright blue/

NURSE 1: I think it was minus three the first day that we were out? But it didn't matter. The atmosphere when we were there/

NURSE 2: /it was very much a sense of togetherness.

NURSE 3: People were just buzzing.

NURSE 1: You wouldn't be aware that you were stood there for six hours.

NURSE 2: (*Wistfully*) There were some beautiful signs/

NURSE 3: /My friend had a sign that said "nobody likes the clap"

NURSE 2: People brought dogs, people brought kids/

NURSE 3: /And despite what you'd see on the news, we never felt like we didn't have support from people.

NURSE 2: It was really nice.

NURSE 1: I was proud of our profession, people were just standing up for themselves/

NURSE 2: /And like the day where we marched down to the bus garage, where the bus drivers were also on strike, and then the bus drivers marched up to join us.

NURSE 1: Everyone was excited,you know, like what's gonna come out of this?

NURSE 3: The reason why nurses are striking and fighting for the NHS is because you've been trained to care for people at a certain level and you can't.

NURSE 2: There's no way it's feasible for it to carry on as it is. We see it, we say it, but no one listens.

NURSE 1: Like, you wouldn't have an F1 team with only two members of staff to do the wheel changing, do you know what I mean? It just wouldn't work. But that's the situation that we're in.

NURSE 3: With striking, if you work in the post office, the worst thing that happens is that someone won't get their post. Trainlines? The trains will be late and you might not get somewhere on time. When we strike, when junior doctors strike, when radiologists strike, people die.

NURSE 2: I mean... I heard mutterings of people who'd be like, oh I don't think it's right. What about the patients who you know might die?

NURSE 1: It's so hard because you're in a profession where you're trying to stop people from dying or make their death as nice as possible.

NURSE 3: I was like, but you see people die all the time. How many times have you had someone that's been end of life on your ward that you've not been able to see them for a shift because you're too busy?

NURSE 2: Too many.

NURSE 1: We had someone die in the chair in the waiting area, and unfortunately, that's not the first time in 12 months. And that's not the first time in the past two weeks either.

NURSE 2: I think you suffer quite a lot of moral injury when you're working in an organisation and having to uphold, uphold like a level of care that you don't think is/

NURSE 3: /Patients aren't dying because nurses are striking, nurses are striking because patients are dying.

NURSE 1: I think it's still worth fighting and pushing. Always.

SCENE 14

A kettle boils. A breath. Perhaps one nurse makes tea for the other two. Each takes comfort from their first sip.

NURSE 2: I think I'll always be a nurse. Probably. As much as some days I think "I'm just gonna quit", I don't think I'll ever actually do it.

NURSE 1: I don't know.
When you do get that feedback, when people actually say thank you? Properly? You don't get it very often and especially where I work you don't get cards and stuff. But there's been times when people have, and you know it just makes you feel like actually, maybe I'm actually doing OK.

NURSE 2: You're so burnt out, you're just like OK we've got to keep it moving. And there are days. But then you catch yourself, you remember the responsibility that you've been given.
It's such an important thing. You're just like... breathe, have a breather. They need you, the patients need you.

NURSE 1: I'll speak about some things to some of my friends and they'll be like, oh my God, like, how'd you deal with that? And I was like, uh, I wasn't in for that reaction. I just wanted to. Kind of voice it out.

NURSE 2: It becomes so much a part of your identity. Of who you are.

NURSE 1: I've not had a relationship with someone that wasn't a nurse since well, since 2016, 17? And I started in healthcare in 2014. Because I think no one else, or like people that aren't in, either shift work or emergency services, kind of... I don't know.

NURSE 3: I stopped nursing like a year ago. So it feels quite distant because of that.

NURSE 1: I did a campaign for male nursing, and they still now try and get me to do these things going around to schools, trying to encourage young people into healthcare and whatnot. But I dunno anymore?

NURSE 3: When I think about those memories, they definitely feel less rushed than they used to. I feel like the adrenaline has finally left my body. Finally.

NURSE 2: It's like, your life. It's so hard to stop being that person.

NURSE 3: It feels so important as well to have a purpose, and then all of a sudden finding a new purpose is really strange. You're sort of just like /

NURSE 2: /Floating.

NURSE 3: Yeah, floating all of a sudden. And I kept promising myself. Like, you're going to do the course and it's gonna be better, it's gonna be better. You're gonna be able to manage it and you're gonna feel like... sure of yourself again. But like, the person who did all those things just feels so far away now?

NURSE 1: It sort of feels like an addiction. It feels really strange to be without that fast-paced, urgent world.

NURSE 2: You see so much love it's amazing. And so much tenderness. But you also see so much sadness, it's very hard to not carry a small part of that with you, I think, forever.

NURSE 3: It's alarming to suddenly leave it and be like I don't do that anymore. But then, I did work in Intensive Care.

NURSE 1: You just hope it's all worth it, don't you. You hope it is.

Long Pause.

A breath.

Sorry I don't know if I'm saying the right thing.

SCENE 15

NURSE 3: I was dead set against nursing. My Mum's a nurse as well and I didn't wanna be like my Mum. That's what you're like when you're a teenager. I remember thinking: I wanna be a PE teacher.

NURSE 1: Patients don't care if they get their drugs on time, if their observations are alright. They care if you know how they like their cup of tea. Do you know what I mean?

NURSE 2: Watching them strapping these babies to themselves and just running. I just couldn't comprehend the human capacity to go so far. So that got me thinking.

Pause.

The lighting changes suddenly. NURSE 3 and NURSE 1 look to comfort NURSE 2.

NURSE 2: There was this girl, 15, And she was very tall, like very tall.
I remember she took up the whole bed. She had this fiery red hair. She wasn't my patient. But she came on my shift, so I was helping get the bed space ready.
The paramedics had found her under a train. Folded in half. And all her skin had come off. But she was alive.
I felt very conflicted. She had been on day release from this like, assisted living for people that were suffering quite severely from mental health issues.
And she'd gone to visit her family and then gone to the tube and tried to kill herself.

I just remember being like... I dunno if we've done the right thing. I thought: this is very much a person who does not want to be on this planet anymore? Um, and I found it very difficult. Like I found, I became very emotional.

It was a long process. Very small steps. But she improved and eventually stepped down from intensive care. She got a place in a proper rehab hospital.

I didn't think I'd ever hear anything from it. But I was like always thinking about her.

And then I came in one day and she'd sent the unit a letter. It was like, I don't remember much from like that time. I don't really remember it being in that place, but like, I want to be a nurse now. I want to be a nurse now.

And I was like, oh my God. Oh, fuck.

BLACKOUT.

ALSO AVAILABLE FROM SALAMANDER STREET

All Salamander Street plays can be bought in bulk at a discount for performance or study. Contact info@salamanderstreet.com to enquire about performance licenses.

TRADE by Ella Dorman-Gajic
ISBN: 9781914228865

Exploring the currency of female bodies in an underground world, Ella Dorman-Gajic's Trade powerfully pulls into question the archetype of the "perfect female victim" by examining the psychology of a morally complex protagonist.

SHE by Anthony Clark
ISBN: 9781739103057

Seven short plays charting the experiences of different women from childhood to old age, these stories, each with an intriguing twist, are visceral, poignant and laced with humour.

ALGORITHMS by Sadie Clark
ISBN: 9781738429394

A bisexual Bridget Jones for the online generation.

these words that'll linger like ghosts till the day i drop down dead by Georgie Bailey
ISBN: 9781914228896

An experimental play about dealing with grief and mental health crises by award-winnning playwright

THE NOBODIES by Amy Guyler
ISBN: 9781914228100

A dark, political thriller about inequality and social discontent. Winner of the Common Award.

COWBOYS AND LESBIANS by Billie Esplen
ISBN: 9781914228902

A queer romantic comedy which examines the intersection between sexuality and fantasy through the eyes of two closeted teenage girls.

www.salamanderstreet.com

www.ingramcontent.com/pod-product-compliance
Lightning Source LLC
Chambersburg PA
CBHW070034110426
42741CB00035B/2773